DIET PATH TO HEALTHY AGING

Nourishing Your Body and Mind for Lifelong Vitality

Pamela Biggs

Table of Content

Introduction

Welcome to "Diet Path To Longevity and Healthy Aging: Nourishing Your Body and Mind for Lifelong Vitality." In this book, we will explore the profound impact that nutrition has on promoting longevity and overall well-being. We live in a time where people are increasingly seeking ways to enhance their health and extend their lifespan. While genetics and lifestyle factors play a role, the choices we make regarding what we eat have a significant influence on our health, vitality, and how we age.

The purpose of this book is to provide you with valuable insights and practical guidance on optimizing your nutrition to support a vibrant and fulfilling life. We will delve into the essential nutrients your body needs as you age, explore the power of antioxidants in combating age-related damage, and discuss the critical role of your gut microbiome in promoting longevity.

You will also discover the benefits of various dietary patterns, including the Mediterranean diet and plant-based approaches, and learn how intermittent fasting and caloric restriction can positively impact your health and lifespan. We will delve into the topic of inflammation and provide you with strategies to control chronic inflammation through proper nutrition.

Additionally, we will introduce you to a range of superfoods and nutritional powerhouses that can provide exceptional health benefits, as well as explore the vital connection between nutrition and cognitive health. Lastly, we will touch upon the environmental impact of our food choices and the importance of sustainable eating practices.

Throughout this book, you will find evidence-based information, practical tips, and delicious recipes to help you incorporate optimal nutrition into your daily life. By making informed choices and nourishing your body with the right foods, you can embark on a journey of improved health, enhanced vitality, and longevity.

To illustrate the transformative power of optimal nutrition, let me share with you the story of Sarah.

Sarah, a vibrant woman in her early 60s, had always been passionate about living a healthy lifestyle. She exercised regularly, maintained a positive mindset, and was mindful of her dietary choices. However, as she entered her 50s, she noticed that her energy levels were declining, and she began experiencing age-related health concerns.

Determined to regain her vitality, Sarah decided to delve deeper into the world of nutrition and its influence on aging. She educated herself about the essential nutrients her body needed and discovered the significant role that antioxidants play in combating age-related damage. Sarah made a conscious effort to incorporate more antioxidant-rich foods into her meals, such as colorful fruits and vegetables, nuts, and seeds.

As she continued her journey, Sarah learned about the vital connection between gut health and longevity. She realized that nurturing her gut microbiome through proper nutrition was crucial for her overall well-being. She began incorporating prebiotic-rich foods, such as fiber-rich whole grains and fermented foods like yogurt and sauerkraut, into her daily diet.

Sarah also explored different dietary patterns that promote longevity, including the Mediterranean diet and intermittent fasting. She found joy in creating delicious meals that were not only nourishing but also supported her overall health and vitality.

Over time, Sarah noticed remarkable changes in her well-being. Her energy levels soared, and she felt a renewed sense of vibrancy. She experienced fewer age-related health concerns and noticed improvements in her cognitive function. Sarah's journey with optimal nutrition not only transformed her physical health but also revitalized her outlook on life.

Inspired by her transformation, Sarah began sharing her knowledge and experiences with others. She became an advocate for optimal nutrition, empowering individuals of all ages to make informed choices that would support their well-being and promote longevity.

Sarah's story serves as a powerful reminder that we can shape our health and future through the choices we make every day. By embracing optimal nutrition and fueling our bodies with the right foods, we can unlock our full potential for a vibrant, fulfilling, and long life.

In the pages that follow, we will delve into the science, strategies, and practical tips to help you embark on your transformative journey. Let us explore the path to optimal nutrition for longevity together, empowering you to fuel your body with vibrant life and embrace the incredible possibilities that lie ahead.

So, let us begin this exciting exploration of optimal nutrition for longevity, empowering you to fuel your body with vibrant life and unlock your full potential for a thriving future.

Chapter One

Foundations of Longevity Nutrition

The significance of nutrition in promoting longevity cannot be overstated. Our dietary choices play a pivotal role in determining the quality and quantity of our lives. Nutrition provides the essential building blocks for our cells, tissues, and organs to function optimally. It supplies the necessary nutrients, vitamins, minerals, and antioxidants that support vital bodily processes and help combat age-related damage. By adopting a nutritionally balanced diet, we can enhance our overall health, strengthen our immune system, reduce the risk of chronic diseases, and ultimately increase our chances of living a longer and healthier life. Nutrition is not just about nourishing our bodies; it is a powerful tool that empowers us to take charge of our well-being, unlock our potential for longevity, and embrace a future filled with vitality and vitality.

In addition to supporting our overall health, nutrition also plays a crucial role in mitigating the effects of aging. As we age, our bodies experience natural wear and tear, and we become more susceptible to age-related conditions and diseases. However, a well-balanced and nutrient-rich diet can help slow down the aging process and reduce the risk of age-related ailments.

Nutrition has a profound impact on key biological processes associated with aging, such as cellular repair, DNA stability, inflammation regulation, and oxidative stress management. By consuming a diet rich in antioxidants, phytochemicals, and essential nutrients, we can protect our cells from damage, promote their repair, and maintain their optimal functioning. These nutritional components found in fruits, vegetables, whole grains, lean proteins, and healthy fats contribute to the overall health of our body systems and help preserve our vitality as we age.

Moreover, nutrition influences important factors that contribute to longevity, such as maintaining a healthy weight, managing blood sugar levels, and supporting cardiovascular health. A balanced diet can help prevent obesity, type 2 diabetes, heart disease, and other chronic conditions that can shorten our lifespan. By fueling our bodies with nutrient-dense foods and avoiding excessive consumption of processed foods, added sugars, and unhealthy fats, we can promote metabolic health, regulate hormone levels, and reduce the risk of age-related health complications.

It is important to note that nutrition is not a magic solution to eternal youth, but rather a key component of a holistic approach to healthy aging. Alongside regular physical activity, stress management, and other lifestyle factors, nutrition forms a solid foundation for longevity. By adopting lifelong healthy eating habits, we have the power to optimize our health, slow down the aging process, and increase our chances of enjoying a vibrant and fulfilling life well into our later years.

In the following chapters of this book, we will delve deeper into the specific nutrients, dietary patterns, and strategies that can promote longevity and provide practical guidance on incorporating them into our daily lives. Let us embark on this journey together, empowering ourselves with the knowledge and tools to make informed nutritional choices and unlock the potential for a long, vibrant, and fulfilling life.

The significance of nutrition in promoting longevity

The significance of nutrition in promoting longevity is paramount. Our diet and nutritional choices have a profound impact on our overall health and well-being, directly influencing our ability to live a long and vibrant life. Nutrition provides the essential nutrients, vitamins, minerals, and antioxidants that our bodies require to function optimally and maintain cellular health.

A well-balanced and nutrient-rich diet is crucial for supporting vital bodily processes, such as metabolism, immune function, and DNA repair. It helps to strengthen our immune system, reducing the risk of chronic diseases and infections that can impact our lifespan. By consuming a variety of nutrient-dense foods, including fruits, vegetables, whole grains, lean proteins, and healthy fats, we provide our bodies with the necessary fuel to thrive and flourish.

Proper nutrition also plays a key role in managing and preventing age-related conditions. Certain nutrients and dietary patterns have been associated with a lower risk of chronic diseases, such as heart disease, diabetes, and certain types of cancer. By adopting a healthy eating plan, we can mitigate the risk factors associated with these diseases and promote longevity.

Furthermore, nutrition is closely linked to maintaining a healthy weight and managing body composition. Excess weight and obesity are known risk factors for various health issues, including cardiovascular disease, joint problems, and metabolic disorders. By practicing portion control, choosing nutrient-dense foods, and incorporating regular physical activity, we can maintain healthy body weight and reduce the risk of obesity-related complications.

In addition to physical health, nutrition also plays a crucial role in supporting cognitive function and mental well-being. Certain nutrients, such as omega-3 fatty acids, antioxidants, and B vitamins, have been shown to have a positive impact on brain health and may help reduce the risk of cognitive decline and neurodegenerative diseases.

It is important to recognize that nutrition is not a standalone solution but works in synergy with other lifestyle factors, such as regular exercise, stress management, and adequate sleep, to promote longevity. By adopting a holistic approach that includes a well-balanced diet, physical activity, and other healthy habits, we can optimize our overall health, enhance our quality of life, and increase our chances of enjoying a long and fulfilling journey through the years.

Understanding the impact of dietary choices on health and aging

The impact of dietary choices on health and aging is crucial for promoting optimal well-being. Our food choices play a significant role in shaping our overall health and can greatly influence the aging process.

The nutrients found in our diets, such as carbohydrates, proteins, fats, vitamins, and minerals, have specific roles in supporting bodily functions and maintaining vitality. Adequate intake of these nutrients is essential for cellular repair, energy production, immune function, and other essential processes that contribute to overall health.

Inflammation is a key factor in the aging process and the development of chronic diseases. Certain dietary choices, such as a diet high in processed foods, sugar, and unhealthy fats, can promote inflammation in the body. On the other hand, a diet rich in fruits, vegetables, whole grains, and healthy fats can help reduce inflammation and protect against age-related diseases.

Oxidative stress is another mechanism that contributes to aging and cellular damage. Antioxidants, which are abundant in plant-based foods, help neutralize harmful free radicals and reduce oxidative stress. Consuming a diet rich in colorful fruits and vegetables, as well as nuts, seeds, and whole grains, provides a wide array of antioxidants that can support healthy aging.

Blood sugar control is also important for promoting longevity. Diets high in refined carbohydrates and sugary foods can lead to unstable blood sugar levels, insulin resistance, and an increased risk of chronic diseases. Choosing complex carbohydrates, and fiber-rich foods, and balancing macronutrients can help regulate blood sugar levels and support healthy aging.

Gut health is increasingly recognized as a key factor in overall health and longevity. A diverse and balanced diet that includes prebiotic and probiotic-rich foods promotes a healthy gut microbiome. A healthy gut microbiome has been associated with reduced inflammation, improved nutrient absorption, and enhanced immune function.

Furthermore, the impact of dietary choices on health and aging extends beyond physical well-being to include cognitive function and mental health. Research suggests that certain nutrients, such as omega-3 fatty acids, antioxidants, and B vitamins, play a vital role in brain health and may help reduce the risk of age-related cognitive decline and neurodegenerative diseases like Alzheimer's. Conversely, diets high in saturated fats, refined sugars, and processed foods have been associated with cognitive impairment and an increased risk of mental health disorders.

In addition to individual nutrients, overall dietary patterns have a significant impact on health and aging outcomes. For example, the Mediterranean diet, which is characterized by an abundance of fruits, vegetables, whole grains, legumes, nuts, and healthy fats like olive oil, has been consistently associated with improved longevity and reduced risk of chronic diseases. Similarly, the DASH (Dietary Approaches to Stop Hypertension) diet, which emphasizes fruits, vegetables, low-fat dairy products, whole grains, lean proteins, and limited sodium intake, has been shown to promote cardiovascular health and reduce the risk of hypertension.

Moreover, the benefits of a healthy diet are not limited to the individual. Studies have shown that communities and cultures that follow traditional dietary patterns, rich in whole, unprocessed foods, have lower rates of chronic diseases and increased longevity. This suggests that the impact of nutrition on health and aging extends beyond personal choices to include broader societal and cultural factors.

It is essential to recognize that dietary choices are just one piece of the puzzle when it comes to healthy aging. Other lifestyle factors, such as regular physical activity, stress management, adequate sleep, and social connection, all play critical roles in promoting overall well-being and longevity. By adopting a holistic approach that encompasses a balanced diet along with these lifestyle factors, we can optimize our health, preserve our vitality, and promote healthy aging throughout our lifespan.

Lastly, the overall dietary pattern and lifestyle factors have a cumulative effect on health and aging. Diets such as the Mediterranean diet, which emphasizes whole foods, plant-based sources, and healthy fats, have been linked to longevity and a reduced risk of chronic diseases. Combining a nutrient-dense diet with regular physical activity, stress management, adequate sleep, and other healthy lifestyle habits can optimize health and promote healthy aging.

By understanding the impact of dietary choices on health and aging, we can make informed decisions about our food intake and lifestyle habits. Incorporating a variety of nutrient-rich foods, reducing processed foods and unhealthy fats, and embracing a balanced and sustainable approach to eating can support our overall health, and vitality, and promote healthy aging.

Essential nutrients for healthy aging

Essential nutrients play a vital role in supporting healthy aging by providing the body with the necessary building blocks for optimal functioning and maintenance. Here are some key nutrients that are particularly important for healthy aging:

Protein: Adequate protein intake is crucial for maintaining muscle mass, strength, and function as we age. It supports tissue repair, immune function, and hormone production. Good sources of protein include lean meats, poultry, fish, dairy products, legumes, and plant-based proteins like tofu and tempeh.

Omega-3 fatty acids: These healthy fats have anti-inflammatory properties and are beneficial for brain health and cardiovascular function. They can be found in fatty fish (such as salmon, sardines, and mackerel), flaxseeds, chia seeds, walnuts, and algae-based supplements.

Calcium and Vitamin D: These are nutrients that are essential for reducing the risk of osteoporosis and fractures and maintaining bone health. Calcium-rich foods include dairy products, leafy green vegetables, and fortified plant-based milk alternatives. Vitamin D can be obtained from sunlight exposure and dietary sources like fatty fish, egg yolks, and fortified foods.

Fiber: Adequate fiber intake promotes digestive health, helps regulate blood sugar levels, and supports heart health. whole grains, fruits, vegetables, legumes, nuts, and seeds are good sources of Fibre.

Antioxidants: Antioxidants help protect cells from damage caused by free radicals, which can contribute to aging and chronic diseases. Colorful fruits and vegetables, berries, nuts, and green tea are excellent sources of antioxidants.

B vitamins: B vitamins, including B12, B6, and folate, are essential for energy production, brain health, and the formation of red blood cells. Sources of B vitamins include meat, fish, poultry, eggs, dairy products, legumes, leafy greens, and fortified cereals.

Magnesium: Magnesium is involved in hundreds of enzymatic reactions in the body and plays a role in maintaining bone health, muscle function, and cardiovascular health. Excellent sources of magnesium include legumes, leafy green vegetables, whole grains, nuts, and seeds.

It is important to note that a balanced and varied diet that includes a wide range of nutrient-dense foods is the best way to obtain these essential nutrients. However, in some cases, dietary supplements may be recommended to ensure adequate intake, especially for certain populations or individuals with specific dietary restrictions or medical conditions. Consulting with a healthcare professional or registered dietitian can provide personalized guidance on meeting nutrient needs for healthy aging.

The role of macronutrients and micronutrients in longevity

Macronutrients and micronutrients both play important roles in promoting longevity and overall health. Let's explore their significance individually:

Macronutrients:

Carbohydrates: Carbohydrates provide the body with energy and are a primary fuel source. Opting for complex carbohydrates, such as whole grains, legumes, and vegetables, over simple carbohydrates helps maintain stable blood sugar levels and provides sustained energy.

Proteins: These are important for producing enzymes and hormones, building and repairing tissues, and supporting immune function. Adequate protein intake is important for preserving muscle mass and strength, which can decline with age. Including lean meats, poultry, fish, dairy products, legumes, and plant-based proteins in the diet can ensure sufficient protein intake.

Fats: Healthy fats, such as monounsaturated and polyunsaturated fats, are crucial for brain function, hormone production, and absorption of fat-soluble vitamins. Healthy fats sources include nuts, avocados, fatty fish, seeds, and olive oil. It is important to moderate the intake of saturated and trans fats, which can contribute to cardiovascular disease.

Micronutrients:

Vitamins: Vitamins are essential for various bodily functions, including energy production, immune support, and cellular maintenance. Examples of key vitamins for longevity include vitamin C (found in citrus fruits and leafy greens), vitamin E (found in nuts, seeds, and vegetable oils), and vitamin D (obtained through sunlight exposure and dietary sources like fatty fish and fortified foods).

Minerals: Minerals play crucial roles in maintaining healthy bodily functions. Calcium and magnesium, for example, support bone health, while iron aids in oxygen transport. Foods like dairy products, leafy greens, nuts, seeds, and lean meats are good sources of these minerals.

Phytochemicals: Phytochemicals are plant compounds that have been linked to various health benefits, including anti-inflammatory and antioxidant effects. They are found in fruits, vegetables, herbs, spices, and other plant-based foods. Examples include lycopene in tomatoes, resveratrol in grapes, and curcumin in turmeric.

It is important to note that maintaining a balanced and varied diet that includes a wide range of whole foods is key to obtaining an optimal mix of macronutrients and micronutrients. Nutritional needs may vary based on individual factors, such as age, sex, activity level, and underlying health conditions. Consulting with a healthcare professional or registered dietitian can help determine specific nutrient requirements and provide personalized recommendations for achieving longevity through proper nutrition.

Importance of hydration for overall well-being

Hydration is of utmost importance for overall well-being as it plays a vital role in maintaining various bodily functions and promoting optimal health. Here are some key reasons why hydration is essential:

Maintaining fluid balance: Water is the main component of our body, accounting for a significant portion of our weight. It is involved in maintaining fluid balance, which is crucial for the proper functioning of cells, tissues, and organs. Adequate hydration helps regulate body temperature, lubricate joints, and support digestion.

Optimal organ function: Staying hydrated is essential for the optimal function of vital organs. Water is needed for the kidneys to filter waste products and toxins from the blood and produce urine. Proper hydration also supports the healthy functioning of the liver, which is responsible for metabolizing nutrients and detoxifying the body.

Physical performance and energy levels: Dehydration can negatively impact physical performance and energy levels. When the body is not adequately hydrated, it may lead to fatigue, decreased endurance, reduced strength, and impaired cognitive function. Maintaining hydration levels is especially important during physical activity to support optimal performance and prevent exercise-related heat illnesses.

Digestion and nutrient absorption: Water plays a key role in digestion and nutrient absorption. It helps break down food, facilitates the transport of nutrients across the digestive system, and supports the smooth movement of waste through the intestines. Sufficient hydration aids in preventing constipation and promoting regular bowel movements.

Skin health and appearance: Hydration is essential for maintaining healthy skin. Proper water intake helps keep the skin hydrated, supple, and less prone to dryness and wrinkles. It also supports the elimination of toxins through sweat, promoting clearer and healthier-looking skin.

Cognitive function and mental well-being: Studies have shown that even mild dehydration can have negative effects on cognitive function, mood, and mental performance. Staying properly hydrated helps enhance concentration, memory, and overall mental clarity.

Regulation of appetite and weight management: Sometimes, thirst can be mistaken for hunger, leading to unnecessary calorie intake. Adequate hydration can help regulate appetite, promote a feeling of fullness, and support weight management efforts.

It is important to note that individual hydration needs may vary depending on factors such as age, activity level, climate, and overall health. It is recommended to drink water throughout the day, listen to your body's thirst signals, and consume additional fluids during periods of increased physical activity or in hot weather.

In conclusion, maintaining proper hydration is crucial for overall well-being. By drinking an adequate amount of water and staying hydrated, we can support bodily functions, promote optimal physical and mental performance, and contribute to our overall health and vitality.

Chapter Two

Anti-Aging Antioxidants

Anti-aging antioxidants play a crucial role in combating the effects of aging and promoting overall health and well-being. As we age, our bodies are exposed to various factors that can accelerate the aging process, such as oxidative stress, free radicals, and environmental toxins. Antioxidants, which are naturally occurring compounds found in certain foods and supplements, have the remarkable ability to neutralize free radicals and protect against cellular damage.

The term "anti-aging antioxidants" refers to a diverse group of compounds that help counteract the effects of oxidative stress on the body. They work by stabilizing free radicals, which are highly reactive molecules that can damage cells, proteins, and DNA. By neutralizing free radicals, antioxidants help reduce the risk of age-related diseases and promote a more youthful appearance.

In addition to their role in neutralizing free radicals, anti-aging antioxidants also support cellular repair mechanisms, promote collagen synthesis, and protect against UV damage. These benefits contribute to smoother skin, improved skin texture and tone, and a reduction in the appearance of wrinkles and fine lines.

While antioxidants are naturally produced in the body, their levels can decline with age, making it essential to obtain them through a balanced diet or supplementation. Fruits, vegetables, nuts, seeds, and certain beverages like green tea are rich sources of antioxidants. Incorporating these antioxidant-rich foods into our daily routine can help optimize the benefits and promote overall health and longevity.

In this chapter, we will explore the mechanisms of action of anti-aging antioxidants, their specific benefits for the skin and overall health, food sources that are high in antioxidants, and tips for incorporating them into our lifestyle. Understanding the power of anti-aging antioxidants can empower us to make informed choices that support healthy aging and maintain a youthful appearance.

Common Antioxidant

Here are some important anti-aging antioxidants:

Vitamin C: This water-soluble vitamin is a potent antioxidant that helps protect against oxidative stress. It supports collagen synthesis, which promotes skin elasticity and reduces the appearance of wrinkles. Vitamin C is found in citrus fruits, berries, kiwis, bell peppers, and leafy greens.

Vitamin E: Vitamin E is a fat-soluble antioxidant that protects cell membranes from oxidative damage. It also helps maintain healthy skin and supports immune function. Sources of vitamin E include nuts, seeds, vegetable oils, and leafy greens.

Beta-carotene: Beta-carotene is a precursor to vitamin A and a powerful antioxidant. It helps protect against sun damage, supports eye health, and promotes healthy skin. Beta-carotene is found in orange and yellow fruits and vegetables, such as carrots, sweet potatoes, and apricots.

Selenium: Selenium is a mineral that works as a cofactor for antioxidant enzymes, helping to neutralize free radicals. It also supports thyroid function and immune health. Good sources of selenium include Brazil nuts, seafood, poultry, and whole grains.

Coenzyme Q10 (CoQ10): CoQ10 is an antioxidant that plays a role in energy production within cells. It helps protect against oxidative damage and supports heart health. CoQ10 is naturally present in small amounts in certain foods like fish, meat, and whole grains. It can also be taken as a supplement.

Resveratrol: Resveratrol is a naturally occurring compound found in red grapes, berries, and peanuts. It has been shown to have antioxidant and anti-inflammatory properties and may help protect against age-related diseases.

Polyphenols: Polyphenols are a group of antioxidants found in a variety of plant-based foods, including fruits, vegetables, tea, coffee, and dark chocolate. They have been linked to numerous health benefits, including anti-aging effects.

It's important to note that while antioxidants have shown promise in supporting healthy aging, their effects may vary depending on factors such as dosage, bioavailability, and individual health status. It is generally recommended to obtain antioxidants through a varied and balanced diet that includes a wide range of fruits, vegetables, whole grains, nuts, and seeds. Consult with a healthcare professional or registered dietitian for personalized advice on incorporating antioxidants into your diet and determining the most suitable approach for your specific needs.

Mechanisms of Action of Anti-Aging Antioxidant

The mechanism of action for anti-aging antioxidants involves their ability to counteract the harmful effects of free radicals, enhance cellular repair processes, and preserve the health and functionality of cells and tissues. Here's a detailed explanation of these mechanisms:

Neutralizing Free Radicals: Free radicals are highly reactive molecules that can damage cells and contribute to the aging process. They are produced naturally in the body as byproducts of various metabolic processes, but their levels can increase due to factors like environmental pollutants, UV radiation, and unhealthy lifestyle habits. Antioxidants help neutralize free radicals by donating an electron to stabilize them. This process prevents free radicals from causing oxidative damage to cellular components, including DNA, proteins, and lipids.

Enhancing Cellular Repair: Antioxidants play a crucial role in cellular repair mechanisms, promoting the restoration and maintenance of healthy cells. They support DNA repair processes, which are essential for maintaining the integrity of the genetic material and preventing mutations that can lead to premature aging. Antioxidants also facilitate cell regeneration and renewal, helping to replace damaged or old cells with new ones. Furthermore, they support mitochondrial function, the energy-producing powerhouses of cells, which can decline with age.

Preserving Collagen and Elasticity: Collagen and elastin are proteins that provide structural support and elasticity to the skin, helping to maintain a youthful appearance. However, their production and quality can decline with age due to various factors, including oxidative stress. Antioxidants help protect collagen and elastin fibers by reducing oxidative damage and supporting the synthesis of new collagen. This helps to preserve skin elasticity and reduce the appearance of wrinkles and fine lines.

By neutralizing free radicals, enhancing cellular repair processes, and preserving collagen and elasticity, anti-aging antioxidants can promote healthier and more youthful-looking skin, as well as contribute to overall health and longevity.

It's important to note that the effectiveness of antioxidants in combating aging depends on various factors, including the specific antioxidant, its concentration, and the overall lifestyle and environmental factors that contribute to oxidative stress. A balanced diet rich in fruits, vegetables, and other antioxidant-rich foods, along with a healthy lifestyle, can optimize the benefits of anti-aging antioxidants.

Benefits of Anti-Aging Antioxidants

Reducing Wrinkles and Fine Lines: One of the primary benefits of anti-aging antioxidants is their ability to reduce the appearance of wrinkles and fine lines. Free radicals, which are generated by factors like sun exposure, pollution, and stress, can damage the skin's collagen and elastin fibers. Skin collagen provides structural support, while elastin maintains the skin's elasticity. When these proteins are compromised, the skin becomes less firm and more prone to wrinkles and fine lines. Antioxidants neutralize free radicals, preventing them from causing oxidative damage to the skin's structural components. This helps to preserve collagen and elastin, leading to smoother and more youthful-looking skin.

Improving Skin Texture and Tone: Antioxidants can also improve skin texture and tone. They promote cell regeneration and renewal, which helps to slough off dead skin cells and reveal fresh, healthier skin underneath. This process can improve the overall texture of the skin, making it smoother and more even. Additionally, antioxidants have anti-inflammatory properties, which can help reduce redness, irritation, and blotchiness, leading to a more balanced and even skin tone.

Protecting Against UV Damage: UV radiation from the sun is a significant contributor to skin aging. Prolonged and unprotected exposure to the sun's rays can lead to the generation of free radicals and cause oxidative stress in the skin. Antioxidants, particularly those with photoprotective properties like vitamin C and vitamin E, can help neutralize free radicals induced by UV radiation and minimize the damage caused by sun exposure. This can help prevent the formation of sunspots, hyperpigmentation, and other signs of UV-induced skin damage.

Promoting Overall Health and Longevity: Antioxidants are not only beneficial for the skin but also for overall health and longevity. Oxidative stress and free radicals have been linked to various age-related diseases, including cardiovascular disease, neurodegenerative disorders, and certain types of cancer. By reducing oxidative stress and neutralizing free radicals throughout the body, antioxidants help protect against cellular damage and contribute to overall health and well-being. They support the proper functioning of various systems, including the immune system, and help maintain cellular integrity, which can have a positive impact on longevity.

It's important to note that the benefits of anti-aging antioxidants may vary depending on the specific antioxidant compound, its concentration, and the individual's lifestyle and genetic factors. Additionally, while antioxidants can provide significant benefits, they should not be seen as a standalone solution for aging. Adopting a comprehensive approach to skin care, including sun protection, a balanced diet, regular exercise, and a healthy lifestyle, is essential for achieving optimal anti-aging effects.

Food Sources of Anti-Aging Antioxidants

Consuming a diet rich in antioxidant-rich foods is an effective way to support healthy aging and maintain optimal health. Here are some common food sources that are abundant in anti-aging antioxidants:

Fruits and Vegetables:

- Berries (such as blueberries, strawberries, and raspberries)
- Citrus fruits (such as oranges, lemons, and grapefruits)
- Leafy green vegetables (such as spinach, kale, and broccoli)
- Brightly colored fruits and vegetables (such as tomatoes, carrots, and bell peppers)
- Pomegranates
- Grapes

Nuts and Seeds:

- Almonds
- Walnuts
- Flaxseeds
- Chia seeds
- Sunflower seeds

Green Tea:

Green tea is rich in polyphenols, which are powerful antioxidants. It is particularly high in a type of polyphenol called catechins, known for its anti-aging properties.

Dark Chocolate:

Dark chocolate with a high percentage of cocoa (70% or more) contains flavonoids, a type of antioxidant. It's important to choose dark chocolate with minimal added sugar for maximum health benefits.

Other food sources of antioxidants include red wine, beans, whole grains, spices (such as turmeric and cinnamon), and certain herbs (such as oregano and basil).

Incorporating a variety of these antioxidant-rich foods into your diet can provide a wide range of beneficial compounds that help neutralize free radicals and support healthy aging. Aim for a colorful and diverse plate, including a mix of fruits, vegetables, nuts, and seeds, to ensure you're getting a good intake of anti-aging antioxidants.

Lifestyle Tips for Maximizing Antioxidant Benefits

In addition to incorporating antioxidant-rich foods into your diet, certain lifestyle choices can maximize the benefits of antioxidants and promote healthy aging. Here are some detailed explanations of lifestyle tips for maximizing antioxidant benefits:

Eating a Balanced Diet: A well-balanced diet that includes a variety of fruits, vegetables, whole grains, lean proteins, and healthy fats provides a wide array of antioxidants, vitamins, and minerals. Aim to consume a rainbow of colorful fruits and vegetables to ensure you're getting a diverse range of antioxidants. Additionally, opt for minimally processed foods and limit your intake of added sugars and unhealthy fats, as they can contribute to oxidative stress and counteract the benefits of antioxidants.

Regular Exercise: Engaging in regular physical activity has been shown to enhance antioxidant defenses in the body. Exercise promotes blood circulation, oxygen delivery, and the production of endogenous antioxidants, such as glutathione. Aim for a combination of cardiovascular exercises, strength training, and flexibility exercises to maximize the benefits for your overall health and well-being.

Managing Stress Levels: Chronic stress can lead to increased oxidative stress in the body. Finding healthy ways to manage stress, such as practicing relaxation techniques (e.g., deep breathing, meditation, yoga), engaging in hobbies, and spending time with loved ones, can help reduce stress levels and support a healthier antioxidant balance.

Getting Sufficient Sleep: Quality sleep is essential for overall health and optimal functioning of antioxidant defense systems. During sleep, the body repairs and regenerates cells, including those involved in antioxidant defenses. Aim for 7-9 hours of restful sleep each night to support your body's natural antioxidant processes.

Limiting Exposure to Environmental Toxins: Minimizing exposure to environmental toxins, such as air pollution, cigarette smoke, and harmful chemicals, can help reduce oxidative stress. Whenever possible, avoid smoking and secondhand smoke, choose natural and non-toxic household products, and minimize exposure to pollutants by improving indoor air quality.

Avoiding Excessive Alcohol Consumption: Excessive alcohol consumption can lead to increased oxidative stress and damage to cells and tissues. Limit your alcohol intake to moderate levels (up to one drink per day for women and up to two drinks per day for men) or consider abstaining altogether to support antioxidant balance and overall health.

Maintaining a Healthy Weight: Maintaining a healthy weight through a balanced diet and regular exercise can help optimize antioxidant benefits. Excess body weight and obesity have been associated with increased oxidative stress and inflammation. By achieving and maintaining a healthy weight, you can reduce the burden of oxidative stress on your body and promote a more balanced antioxidant status.

By adopting these lifestyle tips, you can maximize the benefits of antioxidants in your body and support healthy aging. Remember that consistency and a holistic approach to wellness are key to reaping the full potential of antioxidants in maintaining optimal health and well-being.

Chapter Three

Nurturing Your Microbiome for Longevity

Nurturing your microbiome for longevity has emerged as a key strategy in promoting overall health and extending our lifespan. The human microbiome, consisting of trillions of microorganisms residing within our bodies, plays a vital role in various physiological processes, including digestion, immune function, and metabolism. By fostering a healthy and diverse microbiome, we can positively impact our longevity and enhance our overall well-being.

Scientific research has shed light on the profound influence of the microbiome on age-related conditions, such as cardiovascular disease, neurodegenerative disorders, and metabolic disorders. It has become clear that the composition and balance of our microbiome are intricately linked to our health outcomes as we age.

Nurturing your microbiome involves implementing lifestyle choices that support a thriving microbial community. One crucial aspect is adopting a diet rich in prebiotic fibers, found in fruits, vegetables, and whole grains, which serve as fuel for beneficial gut bacteria. Additionally, incorporating probiotic-rich foods, such as yogurt and fermented vegetables, can introduce beneficial bacteria into the gut.

Managing stress plays a significant role in maintaining a healthy microbiome. Chronic stress can disrupt the balance of gut bacteria, impacting overall health.

Engaging in stress-reducing practices like meditation, mindfulness, and adequate sleep can positively influence the microbiome and promote longevity.

Regular physical activity has also been linked to a diverse and resilient microbiome. Exercise supports microbial diversity and function, contributing to overall gut health. Finding enjoyable activities and incorporating movement into daily routines can have profound effects on the microbiome and, in turn, longevity.

Avoiding unnccessary antibiotic use, which can disrupt the delicate balance of the microbiome, is another crucial aspect of nurturing its health. Antibiotics should be used judiciously and only when necessary to preserve the diversity and functionality of the microbiome.

By nurturing our microbiome, we can enhance immune function, improve digestion, and mitigate the risk of age-related diseases. The intricate relationship between our microbiome and longevity offers exciting possibilities for interventions that can optimize our health and well-being.

In this chapter, we will explore the significance of the microbiome in promoting longevity, the impact of dietary and lifestyle choices on the microbiome, and practical strategies for nurturing and maintaining a healthy microbial community. Together, we can unlock the potential of our microbiome for longevity and enjoy a life of vitality and wellness

The gut-brain connection and Its Influence on Aging

The gut-brain connection can be defined as the bidirectional communication system between the brain and the gastrointestinal tract (the gut). It involves a complex network of neurons, hormones, and immune cells that allow for constant communication and interaction between these two vital systems. Research has increasingly shown that the gut-brain connection plays a significant role in overall health and can influence the aging process. Here's how the gut-brain connection can impact aging:

Microbiota and Aging: The gut is home to trillions of microorganisms, collectively known as the gut microbiota. These microbes have a profound influence on various aspects of health, including metabolism, immune function, and brain health. As we age, the composition and diversity of the gut microbiota can change, potentially impacting the aging process. An imbalance in the gut microbiota, known as dysbiosis, has been associated with age-related conditions such as cognitive decline, neurodegenerative diseases, and inflammation.

Inflammation and Aging: Chronic low-grade inflammation, known as inflammaging, is a hallmark of aging. The gut microbiota and the integrity of the intestinal barrier play a crucial role in modulating inflammation. An imbalance in gut bacteria can lead to increased intestinal permeability (leaky gut), allowing harmful substances to enter the bloodstream and trigger inflammation. Chronic inflammation can contribute to age-related diseases and accelerate the aging process.

Conversely, a healthy gut microbiota can help maintain a balanced inflammatory response and support healthy aging.

Neurotransmitters and Aging: The gut microbiota can produce neurotransmitters and neuropeptides that influence brain function and mood. For example, gut bacteria produce compounds like serotonin, dopamine, and gamma-aminobutyric acid (GABA), which are important for regulating mood, cognition, and stress responses. Alterations in the gut microbiota composition can affect the production and availability of these neurotransmitters, potentially impacting mental health and cognitive function during aging.

Nutrient Absorption and Brain Health: The gut is responsible for absorbing nutrients from the food we eat.

Proper nutrient absorption is essential for maintaining brain health and preventing age-related cognitive decline. A healthy gut lining and microbiota support efficient nutrient absorption, ensuring an adequate supply of essential nutrients for optimal brain function.

Age-Related Digestive Issues: Aging can be associated with changes in digestion and gut function, including decreased motility and digestive enzyme production. These changes can lead to gastrointestinal symptoms such as bloating, constipation, and nutrient malabsorption. Addressing gut health through proper nutrition, maintaining a diverse gut microbiota, and supporting digestive function can help alleviate these age-related digestive issues.

To support a healthy gut-brain connection and promote healthy aging, it is important to focus on a balanced diet that includes a variety of fiber-rich fruits, vegetables, whole grains, and fermented foods. These foods provide prebiotic fibers that nourish beneficial gut bacteria. Regular exercise, stress management techniques, and adequate sleep also play important roles in maintaining a healthy gut-brain connection and supporting healthy aging.

Promoting a healthy gut microbiome through nutrition

Promoting a healthy gut microbiome through nutrition is crucial for overall health and well-being. Here are some dietary strategies to support a healthy gut microbiome:

Eat a diverse range of plant-based foods: Including a variety of fruits, vegetables, whole grains, legumes, nuts, and seeds in your diet provides a wide array of fibers, vitamins, minerals, and phytochemicals that promote a healthy gut microbiome. Aim for different colors and types of plant-based foods to maximize diversity.

Consume prebiotic-rich foods: Prebiotics are types of dietary fibers that serve as food for beneficial gut bacteria. They help nourish and support the growth of these bacteria. Foods rich in prebiotics include onions, garlic, leeks, asparagus, bananas, oats, and legumes. Including these foods regularly can help promote a healthy gut microbiome.

Include fermented foods: Fermented foods contain beneficial bacteria or yeast that can help populate the gut with healthy microbes. Examples are yogurt, kefir, kimchi, tempeh, and miso. Adding fermented foods to your diet can introduce beneficial probiotics and support a balanced gut microbiome.

Consume adequate dietary fiber: Fiber is essential for a healthy gut. It adds bulk to the stool, supports regular bowel movements, and acts as a food source for beneficial bacteria. Good sources of dietary include whole grains, fruits, vegetables, legumes, and nuts. Aim for the recommended daily intake of fiber (around 25-38 grams for adults).

Limit processed and sugary foods: Highly processed foods and those high in added sugars can negatively impact the gut microbiome. They can promote the growth of less desirable bacteria and reduce the diversity of beneficial microbes. Minimize the consumption of processed snacks, sugary drinks, refined grains, and desserts.

Consume healthy fats: Including sources of healthy fats, such as avocados, nuts, seeds, and olive oil, can support a healthy gut microbiome. These fats help reduce inflammation and provide building blocks for the production of beneficial compounds in the gut.

Stay hydrated: Drinking an adequate amount of water is important for maintaining a healthy gut. It helps keep the digestive system functioning optimally and supports the transport of nutrients to the cells. Aim to drink enough water throughout the day.

Limit antibiotic use when unnecessary: Antibiotics can disrupt the balance of gut bacteria, so it's important to use them judiciously and only when necessary. If you do need to take antibiotics, discuss with your healthcare provider about potential strategies to support gut health during and after the course of antibiotics, such as taking probiotics.

Remember that everyone's gut microbiome is unique, and it may take time to notice the effects of dietary changes on gut health. It's also important to make gradual changes and listen to your body's response. If you have specific dietary concerns or health conditions, it's recommended to consult with a healthcare professional or registered dietitian for personalized advice on promoting a healthy gut microbiome through nutrition.

Prebiotics, probiotics, and fermented foods for gut health

Prebiotics, probiotics, and fermented foods are all beneficial for promoting a healthy gut microbiome. Here's an overview of each:

Prebiotics: Prebiotics are types of dietary fibers that serve as a food source for beneficial bacteria in the gut. They help stimulate the growth and activity of these bacteria, promoting a healthy gut microbiome. Prebiotics pass through the upper gastrointestinal tract undigested and reach the colon, where they are fermented by gut bacteria. This fermentation process produces short-chain fatty acids, which provide energy for the colon cells and support a healthy gut environment.

Common sources of prebiotics include:

- Onions, garlic, leeks, and shallots
- Asparagus
- Jerusalem artichokes
- Chicory root

- Bananas
- Oats
- Barley
- Legumes (beans, lentils, chickpeas)

Including these prebiotic-rich foods in your diet regularly can help nourish beneficial gut bacteria and support a healthy gut microbiome.

Probiotics: Probiotics are live beneficial bacteria or yeasts that, when consumed, can confer health benefits to the host. They help restore and maintain a balanced gut microbiome. They can be found in certain foods or taken as supplements. Common strains of probiotics include Lactobacillus and Bifidobacterium species.

Foods rich in probiotics include:

- Yogurt
- Kefir

- Sauerkraut

- Kimchi

- Miso

- Tempeh

- Kombucha

Consuming these probiotic-rich foods regularly can introduce beneficial bacteria to your gut and support a healthy gut microbiome. Probiotic supplements are also available and can be helpful, especially during and after antibiotic use or for specific gut-related conditions. It's important to choose high-quality probiotic products with strains that have been studied for their health benefits.

Fermented foods: Fermented foods undergo a process of natural fermentation, where beneficial bacteria or yeasts convert sugars into alcohol or organic acids. This process enhances the flavor, texture, and shelf life of the food and can also introduce beneficial microbes. Fermented foods can contain live probiotics or the byproducts of the fermentation process, such as organic acids and enzymes, which can support gut health.

Examples of fermented foods include:

- Yogurt
- Kefir
- Sauerkraut
- Kimchi
- Pickles (made through lacto-fermentation)
- Miso
- Tempeh

Including these fermented foods in your diet can introduce beneficial bacteria and their byproducts to support a healthy gut microbiome.

It's important to note that the effects of prebiotics, probiotics, and fermented foods can vary depending on factors such as the specific strains or types of bacteria involved, individual gut health, and overall diet and lifestyle. For personalized advice on incorporating prebiotics, probiotics, and fermented foods into your diet, it's recommended to consult with a healthcare professional or registered dietitian.

Chapter Four

Dietary Patterns for Longevity

Dietary patterns play a crucial role in determining our health outcomes and influencing the aging process. Research has identified specific dietary patterns that promote longevity, enhance overall health, and reduce the risk of chronic diseases. By adopting these dietary patterns, we can optimize our nutritional intake, support healthy aging, and increase our chances of living a longer, healthier life.

Examining different dietary approaches

Mediterranean Diet:

The Mediterranean diet is widely recognized as one of the healthiest dietary patterns for longevity. It is inspired by the traditional eating habits of people living in countries bordering the Mediterranean Sea. This diet is characterized by high consumption of fruits, vegetables, whole grains, legumes, nuts, and seeds. Olive oil is the primary source of fat, while red meat and processed foods are limited. The Mediterranean diet is rich in antioxidants, fiber, monounsaturated fats, and a variety of essential nutrients. Studies have consistently shown that this dietary pattern is associated with a reduced risk of heart disease, stroke, cognitive decline, and certain cancers. It promotes cardiovascular health, lowers inflammation, supports healthy aging, and provides a wide range of nutrients that contribute to overall well-being.

Plant-Based Diet:

A plant-based diet emphasizes the consumption of plant-derived foods while minimizing or eliminating animal products. It includes an abundance of fruits, vegetables, whole grains, legumes, nuts, and seeds. Plant-based diets are rich in fiber, vitamins, minerals, and phytochemicals, which have been associated with a lower risk of chronic diseases and improved longevity. They provide essential nutrients while reducing the intake of saturated fats and cholesterol found in animal-based products.

Plant-based diets have been linked to a reduced risk of cardiovascular disease, type 2 diabetes, certain cancers, and obesity. They also promote healthy weight management, support gut health, and possess anti-inflammatory properties. Variations of plant-based diets include vegetarian, vegan, and flexitarian approaches, allowing individuals to choose the level of animal product restriction that suits their preferences and health goals.

Okinawan Diet:

The Okinawan diet is based on the traditional eating habits of the elderly population in Okinawa, Japan. Okinawans have one of the highest life expectancies in the world. The Okinawan diet is characterized by a high intake of plant-based foods, including vegetables, legumes, soy products, and whole grains. It also incorporates moderate amounts of fish and seafood, while red meat and processed foods are consumed sparingly. The Okinawan diet is low in calories but rich in nutrients. It provides a wide range of antioxidants, fiber, and essential fatty acids. Studies have shown that this dietary pattern is associated with a reduced risk of chronic diseases, including heart disease, cancer, and age-related conditions. The Okinawan diet promotes healthy weight management, supports cardiovascular health, and offers a variety of nutrients that contribute to longevity.

By adopting these dietary patterns, we can nourish our bodies with essential nutrients, reduce the risk of chronic diseases, and support healthy aging. These dietary approaches focus on whole, nutrient-dense foods, emphasizing plant-based sources and healthy fats while limiting processed and unhealthy options. Incorporating these dietary patterns into our lifestyle can contribute to a longer, healthier, and more vibrant life.

Benefits of intermittent fasting and caloric restriction

Intermittent fasting and caloric restriction are two dietary approaches that have gained attention for their potential health benefits and impact on longevity. Let's explore the benefits of each approach:

Intermittent Fasting:

Intermittent fasting involves cycling between periods of fasting and eating within a specific time window. Here are some benefits associated with intermittent fasting:

Weight Management: Intermittent fasting can be an effective strategy for weight loss and weight management. Limiting the eating window, can lead to a reduced calorie intake and promote fat loss while preserving lean muscle mass.

Improved Insulin Sensitivity: Intermittent fasting has been shown to enhance insulin sensitivity, which is important for regulating blood sugar levels. This can reduce the risk of insulin resistance, type 2 diabetes, and metabolic syndrome.

Enhanced Autophagy: Intermittent fasting stimulates a process called autophagy, where the body clears out damaged cells and proteins. This cellular recycling process has been linked to various health benefits, including reduced inflammation and improved cellular function.

Cardiovascular Health: Intermittent fasting may improve markers of cardiovascular health, such as blood pressure, cholesterol levels, and triglycerides. It has been associated with a reduced risk of heart disease and other cardiovascular conditions.

Brain Health: Some studies suggest that intermittent fasting may have neuroprotective effects, improving brain health and reducing the risk of neurodegenerative diseases like Alzheimer's and Parkinson's.

Caloric Restriction:

Caloric restriction involves reducing daily calorie intake while still meeting essential nutrient needs. Here are some benefits associated with caloric restriction:

Increased Lifespan: Caloric restriction has been shown to extend lifespan in various organisms, including yeast, worms, flies, and rodents. Although more research is needed on humans, caloric restriction is considered a potential strategy for promoting longevity.

Improved Metabolic Health: Caloric restriction can improve metabolic parameters, such as insulin sensitivity, blood lipid levels, and blood pressure. It may reduce the risk of metabolic diseases like type 2 diabetes and metabolic syndrome.

Reduced Inflammation: Caloric restriction has been associated with reduced levels of inflammation in the body. Chronic inflammation is linked to various age-related diseases, and by reducing inflammation, caloric restriction may help mitigate their risk.

Protection Against Age-Related Diseases: Caloric restriction has shown promise in protecting against age-related diseases, including cardiovascular disease, cancer, and neurodegenerative disorders. It may delay the onset and progression of these conditions.

Enhanced Cellular Function: Caloric restriction can improve cellular function by enhancing mitochondrial health, reducing oxidative stress, and improving cellular repair mechanisms.

It's important to note that both intermittent fasting and caloric restriction should be approached with caution and tailored to individual needs. They may not be suitable for everyone, such as those with certain medical conditions or nutritional requirements. Consulting with a healthcare professional or registered dietitian is recommended before embarking on any significant dietary changes.

Overall, intermittent fasting and caloric restriction hold promise for various health benefits, including weight management, improved metabolic health, enhanced cellular function, and potentially extended lifespan. However, further research is needed to fully understand their long-term effects on humans.

Personalizing your nutrition plan for optimal longevity

Personalizing your nutrition plan for optimal longevity involves considering individual factors such as age, sex, activity level, health status, and personal preferences. Here are some key considerations to help tailor your nutrition plan:

Nutrient-Dense Foods: Focus on consuming a variety of nutrient-dense foods that provide essential vitamins, minerals, antioxidants, and phytochemicals. Include a wide range of colorful fruits and vegetables, whole grains, lean proteins, healthy fats, and plant-based sources of protein.

Balanced Macronutrient Intake: Determine the appropriate balance of macronutrients (carbohydrates, proteins, and fats) based on your individual needs and health goals. Consider consulting with a registered dietitian or nutritionist to determine the ideal macronutrient distribution for your specific requirements.

Adequate Protein Intake: Protein is essential for maintaining muscle mass, supporting immune function, and promoting overall health. Ensure you're consuming enough high-quality protein sources such as lean meats, fish, poultry, dairy products, legumes, and plant-based proteins.

Mindful Caloric Intake: Pay attention to your calorie needs based on your age, sex, activity level, and goals. Ensure you're consuming an appropriate amount of calories to maintain a healthy weight, as excess body weight can increase the risk of chronic diseases.

Healthy Fats: Include healthy fats in your diet, such as avocados, nuts, seeds, olive oil, and fatty fish. These fats provide essential fatty acids and help support brain health, heart health, and overall well-being.

__Hydration:__ Stay properly hydrated by drinking adequate amounts of water throughout the day. Water plays a vital role in various bodily functions and supports overall health.

__Individual Considerations:__ Consider any specific dietary needs or restrictions you may have, such as food allergies, intolerances, or medical conditions. Tailor your nutrition plan accordingly to accommodate these factors.

__Regular Physical Activity:__ Incorporate regular exercise and physical activity into your routine, as it complements a healthy diet and promotes longevity. Consult with a healthcare professional or fitness expert to develop an exercise plan suitable for your fitness level and goals.

__Personal Preferences and Cultural Influences:__ Take into account your personal food preferences and cultural influences when designing your nutrition plan. This ensures the sustainability and enjoyment of the chosen dietary approach.

Regular Monitoring and Adjustments: Regularly assess your nutrition plan and make adjustments as needed. This can involve tracking your food intake, monitoring changes in your body composition, and considering any feedback from healthcare professionals.

Remember, personalized nutrition plans should be based on evidence-based recommendations, individual needs, and professional guidance. Working with a registered dietitian or nutritionist can provide valuable insights and support in developing a tailored nutrition plan that promotes optimal longevity and overall health.

Nutritional strategies to support brain health and cognitive function

Maintaining brain health and supporting cognitive function is essential for overall well-being and longevity. Here are some nutritional strategies to support brain health:

Eat a Balanced Diet: Follow a balanced diet that includes a variety of nutrient-rich foods. Focus on consuming fruits, vegetables, whole grains, lean proteins, healthy fats, and low-fat dairy or dairy alternatives. This ensures an adequate intake of essential vitamins, minerals, antioxidants, and other bioactive compounds that support brain health.

Omega-3 Fatty Acids: Include sources of omega-3 fatty acids in your diet, as they play a crucial role in brain health. Fatty fish like salmon, mackerel, and sardines are great sources of omega-3s. Plant-based sources include walnuts, flaxseeds, and chia seeds. Omega-3 fatty acids have been associated with improved cognitive function and a reduced risk of neurodegenerative diseases.

Antioxidant-Rich Foods: Consume foods rich in antioxidants, such as berries (blueberries, strawberries, etc.), dark leafy greens, colorful fruits and vegetables, and nuts. Antioxidants help protect the brain from oxidative stress and inflammation, which are linked to cognitive decline and neurodegenerative diseases.

Curcumin: Incorporate turmeric or curcumin supplements into your diet. Curcumin, a compound found in turmeric, has been studied for its potential to support brain health. It has antioxidant and anti-inflammatory properties and may enhance memory and cognitive function.

B Vitamins: Ensure an adequate intake of B vitamins, including vitamins B6, B12, and folate. These vitamins are involved in the synthesis of neurotransmitters and play a role in cognitive function. Good sources include fortified cereals, legumes, leafy greens, poultry, fish, and eggs.

Mediterranean Diet: Consider following a Mediterranean-style diet, which includes plenty of fruits, vegetables, whole grains, legumes, nuts, seeds, olive oil, and moderate consumption of fish, poultry, and red wine. The Mediterranean diet has been associated with a reduced risk of cognitive decline and neurodegenerative diseases.

Reduce Added Sugars and Processed Foods: Limit your intake of added sugars and processed foods, as excessive consumption may contribute to inflammation and impair brain health.

Stay Hydrated: Ensure adequate hydration by drinking enough water throughout the day. Dehydration can negatively impact cognitive function, so it's important to maintain proper fluid balance.

Moderate Alcohol Consumption: Excessive alcohol intake can have detrimental effects on brain health. It's generally recommended to limit alcohol consumption to one drink per day for women and up to two drinks per day for men.

Regular Physical Activity: Engage in regular physical activity, as it promotes blood flow to the brain and supports overall brain health. Aim for a combination of aerobic exercise and strength training.

Remember, maintaining a healthy lifestyle that includes a balanced diet, regular exercise, adequate sleep, and engaging in mentally stimulating activities is key to supporting brain health and cognitive function. Seek the advice of a healthcare professional or registered dietitian for personalized advice based on your specific needs and health goals.

Chapter Five

Meal Plans and Recipes

Sample weekly meal plans for longevity and vibrant health

Day 1:

Breakfast: Veggie omelet made with egg whites, spinach, tomatoes, and feta cheese.

Lunch: Quinoa salad with roasted vegetables, chickpeas, feta cheese, and a lemon-herb dressing.

Snack: Greek yogurt with a handful of mixed nuts and berries.

Dinner: Baked salmon with steamed asparagus and quinoa pilaf.

Dessert: Fresh fruit salad.

Day 2:

Breakfast: Overnight oats topped with berries, nuts, and a drizzle of honey or maple syrup.

Lunch: Grilled chicken or tofu wrap with mixed greens, tomatoes, cucumbers, and a light yogurt-based dressing.

Snack: Sliced apples or carrots with almond butter or hummus.

Dinner: Lentil curry with mixed vegetables, served over brown rice.

Dessert: Dark chocolate squares.

Day 3:

Breakfast: Whole grain toast with avocado, smoked salmon, and a sprinkle of lemon juice.

Lunch: Lentil soup with a side of mixed green salad and whole grain bread.

Snack: Homemade energy balls made with dates, nuts, and seeds.

Dinner: Grilled chicken breast with roasted sweet potatoes and sautéed green beans.

Dessert: Greek yogurt with a drizzle of honey and chopped almonds.

Day 4:

Breakfast: Smoothie made with mixed berries, spinach, almond milk, and a scoop of protein powder.

Lunch: Salmon or tuna salad with mixed greens, cherry tomatoes, avocado, and a vinaigrette dressing.

Snack: Rice cakes with avocado and smoked salmon.

Dinner: Zucchini noodles with grilled shrimp, cherry tomatoes, and pesto sauce.

Dessert: Baked apple slices with cinnamon and a dollop of Greek yogurt.

Day 5:

Breakfast: Veggie scramble with eggs or egg whites, spinach, bell peppers, onions, and a sprinkle of cheese.

Lunch: Chickpea and vegetable stir-fry with tofu or shrimp, served over brown rice.

Snack: Veggie sticks with guacamole or salsa.

Dinner: Baked tofu with stir-fried broccoli, bell peppers, and brown rice.

Dessert: Chia seed pudding with mixed berries.

Remember to adjust portion sizes and ingredients based on your specific needs and preferences. Feel free to mix and match meals and snacks throughout the week to create a meal plan that works best for you. Additionally, incorporate plenty of water and herbal teas throughout the day to stay hydrated.

Consulting with a registered dietitian can provide further personalized guidance and help tailor a meal plan to your specific dietary needs and goals.

Nourishing recipes featuring longevity-promoting ingredients

Recipe 1: Mediterranean Stuffed Bell Peppers

Ingredients:

4 bell peppers (any color)

1 cup cooked quinoa

1 cup diced tomatoes

1/2 cup chopped Kalamata olives

1/2 cup crumbled feta cheese

1/4 cup chopped fresh parsley

2 tablespoons extra-virgin olive oil

1 tablespoon lemon juice

1 teaspoon dried oregano

Salt and pepper to taste

Instructions:

Preheat the oven to 375°F (190°C).

Cut the tops off the bell peppers and remove the seeds and membranes.

In a bowl, combine the cooked quinoa, diced tomatoes, Kalamata olives, feta cheese, parsley, olive oil, lemon juice, dried oregano, salt, and pepper. Mix well.

Stuff each bell pepper with the quinoa mixture and place them in a baking dish.

Bake for about 25-30 minutes until the peppers are tender and the filling is heated through.

Serve hot and enjoy!

Recipe 2: Turmeric-Ginger Lentil Soup

Ingredients:

1 tablespoon olive oil

1 onion, chopped

2 cloves garlic, minced

1 tablespoon grated fresh ginger

1 teaspoon ground turmeric

1 cup dried red lentils

4 cups vegetable broth

1 cup chopped carrots

1 cup chopped spinach

Juice of 1 lemon

Salt and pepper to taste

Fresh cilantro for garnish (optional)

Instructions:

Heat olive oil in a large pot over medium heat. Add the onion and sauté until softened.

Add the minced garlic, grated ginger, and turmeric. Cook for another minute until fragrant.

Add the red lentils and vegetable broth to the pot. Bring to a boil, then reduce heat and simmer for about 15-20 minutes until the lentils are tender.

Add the chopped carrots and continue simmering for another 10 minutes until the carrots are cooked.

Stir in the chopped spinach and lemon juice. Season with salt and pepper to taste.

Remove from heat and garnish with fresh cilantro if desired.

Serve hot and enjoy this comforting and nourishing soup!

Recipe 3: Berry Chia Pudding

Ingredients:

1/4 cup chia seeds

1 cup unsweetened almond milk (or any other plant-based milk)

1 tablespoon maple syrup or honey

1/2 teaspoon vanilla extract

Fresh mixed berries (strawberries, blueberries, raspberries) for topping

Optional toppings: sliced almonds, shredded coconut

Instructions:

In a bowl, combine the chia seeds, almond milk, maple syrup (or honey), and vanilla extract. Stir well to combine.

Let the mixture sit for about 5 minutes, then stir again to prevent clumping.

Cover the bowl and refrigerate overnight or for at least 4-6 hours to allow the chia seeds to absorb the liquid and thicken.

When ready to serve, give the pudding a good stir. If desired, add a splash of almond milk to achieve the desired consistency.

Divide the chia pudding into serving bowls or jars and top with fresh mixed berries, sliced almonds, and shredded coconut.

Enjoy this delicious and nutrient-packed breakfast or snack!

These recipes incorporate ingredients known for their potential health benefits, including antioxidants, anti-inflammatory compounds, and other nutrients that support longevity and well-being. Feel free to modify the recipes to suit your taste preferences and dietary needs

Tips for meal prepping and making sustainable dietary changes

Meal prepping and making sustainable dietary changes can be key to maintaining a healthy lifestyle. Here are some tips to help you with both:

Plan Ahead: Set aside some time each week to plan your meals and create a grocery list. This will help you stay organized and ensure you have all the necessary ingredients on hand.

Batch Cooking: Consider batch cooking large quantities of staple foods such as grains, proteins, and roasted vegetables. This way, you can easily assemble meals throughout the week by combining these pre-cooked components.

Portion Control: Use portion control techniques to ensure you're eating appropriate serving sizes. Invest in reusable portion containers or use a kitchen scale to measure servings in advance.

Mix and Match: Prepare versatile ingredients that can be used in various dishes. For example, roasted chicken can be used in salads, wraps, or stir-fries. Roasted vegetables can be served as a side dish, added to grain bowls, or used in omelets.

Store Properly: Invest in quality storage containers that are airtight and freezer-safe. Proper storage will help maintain the freshness and quality of your prepped meals.

Mindful Eating: Practice mindful eating by paying attention to your body's hunger and fullness cues. Eat slowly and savor each bite, allowing yourself to fully enjoy the flavors and textures of your meals.

Start Gradually: Instead of making drastic dietary changes all at once, start by incorporating small sustainable changes. For example, gradually increase your intake of fruits and vegetables or replace sugary beverages with water or herbal tea.

Set Realistic Goals: Set achievable and realistic goals for yourself. Make changes that you can comfortably maintain in the long run, rather than following extreme or restrictive diets that may not be sustainable.

Be Adaptable: Be flexible and adaptable with your meal plan. If unexpected events or cravings arise, allow yourself to make adjustments without feeling guilty. Remember that sustainability is about finding balance and enjoying your food choices.

Seek Support: Find a support system that can help keep you motivated and accountable. This could be a friend, family member, or an online community with similar goals and interests.

Celebrate Success: Acknowledge and celebrate your achievements along the way. Whether it's reaching a milestone or sticking to your meal plan for a week, reward yourself with non-food-related treats or activities that bring you joy.

Remember, sustainable dietary changes are about creating a healthy and enjoyable lifestyle that can be maintained in the long term. Find what works best for you and adapt as needed to support your overall well-being and long-term health goals.

Chapter Six

Longevity and the Environment

Longevity and the environment are closely intertwined. The choices we make regarding our lifestyle and consumption habits can have a significant impact on both our health and the health of the planet. Here are some key points highlighting the connection between longevity and the environment:

Sustainable Food Choices: Opting for a diet rich in plant-based foods, such as fruits, vegetables, whole grains, legumes, and nuts, is not only beneficial for our health but also has a lower environmental impact. Plant-based diets tend to require fewer natural resources, produce fewer greenhouse gas emissions, and contribute to biodiversity conservation.

Reduce Food Waste: Minimizing food waste is important for both longevity and environmental sustainability. By planning meals, properly storing food, and repurposing leftovers, we can reduce the amount of food that goes to waste. This helps conserve resources and reduces greenhouse gas emissions associated with food production and disposal.

Sustainable Agriculture: Supporting sustainable agricultural practices, such as organic farming, agroforestry, and regenerative farming methods, helps promote biodiversity, soil health, and water conservation. Sustainable agriculture aims to minimize the use of synthetic chemicals, protect natural ecosystems, and preserve the long-term productivity of the land.

Conscious Consumption: Being mindful of our consumption habits and opting for products that are ethically and sustainably produced can contribute to both personal well-being and environmental preservation. Choosing eco-friendly and fair-trade products, reducing single-use plastics, and supporting companies with environmentally responsible practices can make a positive impact.

Active Transportation: Opting for active transportation methods like walking, cycling, or using public transportation not only promotes physical activity and longevity but also reduces carbon emissions from individual vehicles. It helps improve air quality and reduce traffic congestion, leading to a healthier and more sustainable environment.

Energy Conservation: Implementing energy-saving practices at home, such as using energy-efficient appliances, properly insulating buildings, and utilizing renewable energy sources, contributes to reducing greenhouse gas emissions and mitigating climate change. Conserving energy helps create a more sustainable future for generations to come.

Waste Reduction and Recycling: Engaging in responsible waste management practices, such as recycling, composting, and minimizing single-use items, helps reduce the amount of waste sent to landfills. It conserves resources, minimizes pollution, and supports a circular economy where materials are reused or repurposed.

By recognizing the interdependence between our well-being and the health of the environment, we can make conscious choices that promote both longevity and a sustainable future. Small individual actions, when combined, can have a significant collective impact on creating a healthier planet for current and future generations.

Conclusion

In conclusion, our choices regarding food and nutrition have a profound impact not only on our health and longevity but also on the environment, animal welfare, and social justice. By embracing an approach of conscious eating, we can make ethical and eco-friendly choices that align with our values and contribute to a more sustainable future.

Anti-aging antioxidants play a crucial role in supporting our well-being and promoting longevity. They help protect our cells from damage caused by free radicals, oxidative stress, and inflammation. Incorporating anti-aging antioxidants into our diet through a variety of nutrient-rich foods and supplements can provide numerous benefits, such as reducing the risk of chronic diseases, enhancing skin health, boosting the immune system, and supporting cognitive function.

Additionally, nurturing our microbiome is essential for long-term health and longevity. The gut microbiome influences various aspects of our well-being, including digestion, nutrient absorption, immune function, and even mental health. By adopting practices such as consuming probiotic-rich foods, eating a diverse range of plant-based foods, and minimizing the use of antibiotics, we can promote a healthy and balanced microbiome.

Furthermore, dietary patterns for longevity emphasize the importance of whole, minimally processed foods, such as fruits, vegetables, whole grains, legumes, lean proteins, and healthy fats. These dietary patterns prioritize nutrient density, balance, and moderation to support optimal health and longevity.

Other strategies for promoting longevity include intermittent fasting, caloric restriction, and personalizing our nutrition plan to meet individual needs. These approaches have been shown to enhance cellular repair, improve metabolic health, and extend lifespan.

To support brain health and cognitive function, incorporating specific nutrients such as omega-3 fatty acids, antioxidants, vitamins, and minerals into our diet is important. These nutrients can help protect against cognitive decline, improve memory and focus, and support overall brain health.

Meal prepping, sustainable dietary changes, and making eco-friendly choices are crucial for maintaining a healthy lifestyle and reducing our environmental impact. By planning meals, minimizing food waste, choosing sustainable food sources, and being mindful of our consumption habits, we can contribute to a more sustainable and ethical food system.

In summary, by adopting a conscious approach to our nutrition and lifestyle choices, we can promote both personal longevity and a sustainable future for the planet. Making informed decisions, embracing sustainable practices, and prioritizing the well-being of ourselves and the environment will contribute to a healthier, more ethical, and resilient world for generations to come.